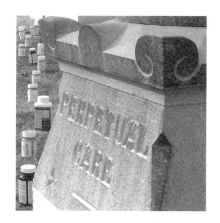

Perpetual Care

For Carol —
Healer, Adventurer, Good friend —
Love Susan

Photographs © 2016 Susan Eisenberg
Cover photograph, *Down This Road*
Author photograph © Estelle Disch
Book design Ilene Horowitz

Library of Congress Cataloging-in-Publication Data

Names: Eisenberg, Susan, 1950- author.
Title: Perpetual care / Susan Eisenberg.
Description: First edition. | Boston, MA : Third Rail Press, 2016.
Identifiers: LCCN 2016001178 | ISBN 9780996131001 (softcover)
Classification: LCC PS3555.I8438 A6 2016 | DDC 811/.54--dc23
LC record available at http://lccn.loc.gov/2016001178

Published by
Third Rail Press
Boston, MA
thirdrailpress@gmail.com

Author contact: www.susaneisenberg.com

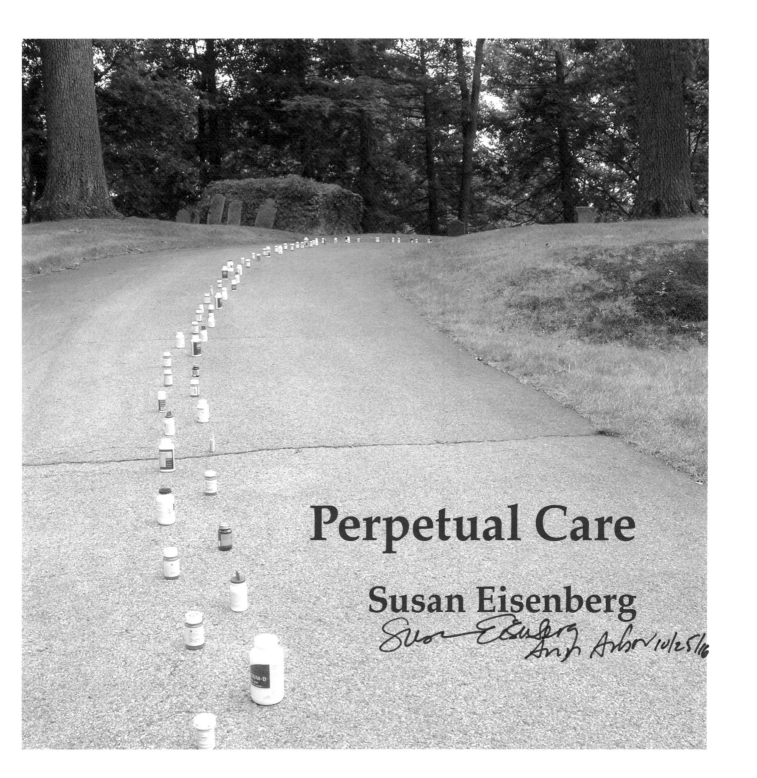

Perpetual Care

Susan Eisenberg

Also by
Susan Eisenberg

Poetry

Blind Spot
Pioneering
It's a Good Thing I'm Not Macho

Nonfiction

We'll Call You If We Need You: Experiences of Women Working Construction

for Rita Arditti
(1934–2009)
dear friend,
guide and grounding rod

Contents

Chief Complaint

Progress Notes

Chief Complaint

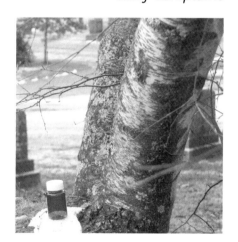

In the Beginning

When pirates commandeered my body
and steered it beyond known maps
into whirlpools
of symptoms that shifted shape

life seemed lost,
spinning in a maelstrom of questions
and tests. And waiting.

What   are you   looking for?

I suppose the nurse meant
not to alarm. She delivered her response
in monotone,
like a tired waitress at a dull
diner listing sandwiches—*tuna, egg salad,*
grilled cheese, ham—no specials
on this menu to excite:
rheumatoid arthritis
HIV
hepatitis
lupus.

But scrawled in the lines of her forehead:
Here be dragons.

Pre-Diagnosis

at first I turn sideways
to slip ahead &
scurry things along

months   seasons   years
time transforms from solid to gas

now I lag   pulling reluctant body parts
through the maze
corridor after corridor   each leading to
another room draped in white paper
where long needles or large mechanical eyes
      probe through my armor
      handing back answers   incomplete
another clue! to hold
this way   that way   even upside-down
might   tell   something

puzzle pieces fingered for edges that interlock
collect in a folder

followed   I am being followed

Confusion

Drifting
        cloudlike

    a flock of words
        from your mouth
  flaps past my ear.

I hear my name.

Driving Home Haiku

Red light. Rest my eyes.
Light's green!—but eyes won't wake up.
Car horns lose patience.

Lupus Outwits Me, Declares Martial Law

Who would dream to awaken from fevered sleep
stun-gunned into paralysis by their own
ruthless doppelganger:
power stations overtaken in a pre-dawn coup;
from every organ of the body
a triumphant, unfamiliar flag!

Who wouldn't be humbled
by their double's brazen brilliance? Or,
begin at once to plot in whispers
the first frantic steps of resistance?

Auto-Immune

Howdumb-isthat?

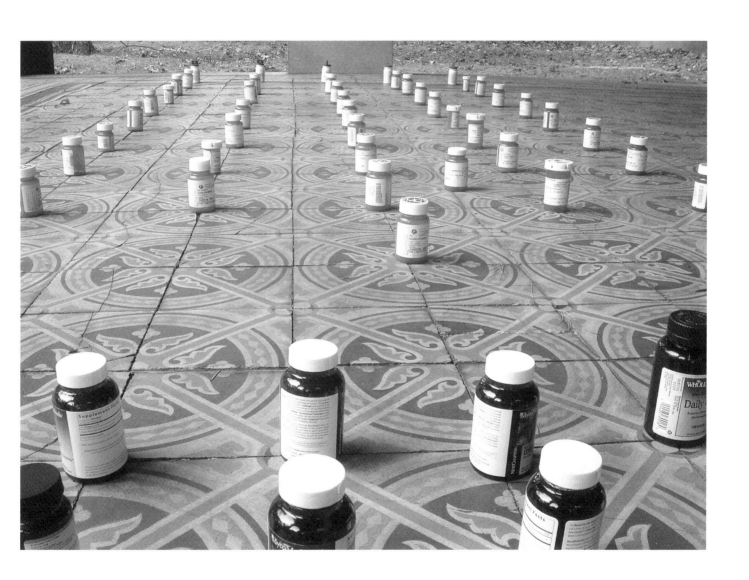

Fatigue

  1) plans
a riptide of exhaustion
pulls my body from land

from my list of to-do's
must-do's . . .

my appointment book:
a tiny dot on shore

  2) physics
gravity
cancels
any will
upright:

limbs
torso
eye-
lids

drain
toward
earth's
core

  3) profile
bossy
stubborn
interrupts
won't cooperate

Chronically Ill

In cell-to-cell combat corporate giants battle
across organs, joints, blood. Knocked
to my knees by the Agri-Industrials, I'm now
acolyte to Big Pharma,
those *liberators*

                        who overstay
and bring their own trouble.
Religiously, on Sunday mornings, I drop
an arsenal of pills into seven plastic boxes—
like a row of miniature coffins.

While faux seeds fall on organic fields,
factories huff and puff, bury and *bye-bye*,
suits reach into bottomless pockets
and toss T-bones to gorge
our three-headed watchdog to sleep.

The soil chokes, fish turn Mad Hatter,
and our booby-trapped bodies implode.

Post-Diagnosis

The doc's wearing a solemn face
as we stroll the gardenpaths of my long chart
to review in methodical detail
our fifteen-year trail: symptoms and tests
now interlocked and named.
At last we reach why he summoned me:

Knife Edge Ridge. Like we're friends
who've aged together meeting over coffee
and he's reached across the table for my hand,
he denies-confirms the abyss:

*Don't live your life like you're sitting
on a ticking time bomb.* Oh, the human condition
in hazardous times. I've swallowed the globe,
our fates entwined.

Disclosure

1)
My mother's frame so tiny,
the bearishness of her hug
surprises. From a woman

who counts each day: *I wish*
I could give you years.

2)
A friend who's heard,
drops by for tea; scans my face
like it's an obituary page.
I hurry him toward World News,
Weather, Living/Arts.

3)
I leave a casual message
about nothing. But in the voice histogram
my daughter deciphers the setback.

I take a bus Boston to New York.
We have lunch.

4)
The woman on the trolley lets the full car
hear her disgust
when my son helps me
take the empty seat
while a pregnant woman stands.

Lupus Conference, Morningstar Baptist Church

Someone will make sure
you have a seat, you have a plate,
you have a raffle ticket
for groceries. Even if you haven't raised
your hand, someone will make sure you speak.
Someone will introduce herself to you;
and you to this one, and another. Yet

this quilt of kindness can't fend off the chill
of why we're here. Like our lives,
the agenda adapts to circumstance:
11:15–11:30 Personal Stories—cancelled.
The speakers on juggling work, family, illness

could not be here. Hospital.

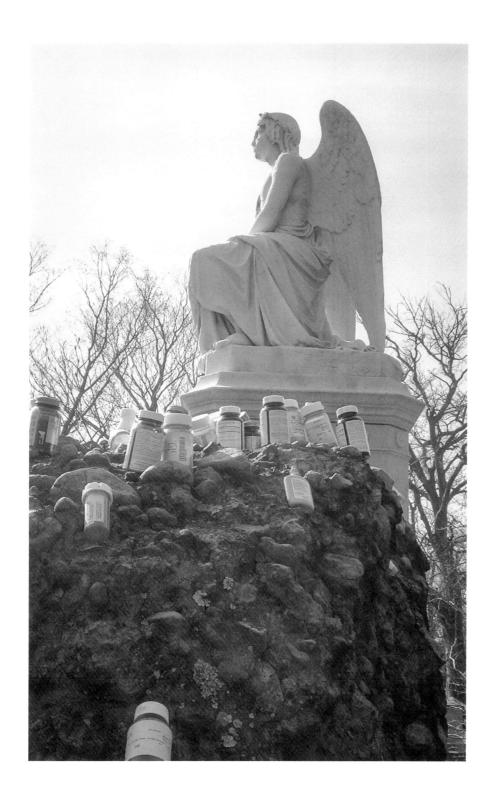

Escape from Prednisone, Second Attempt

Jubilant,
I swim
confident
strokes
toward open
waters

> but Pain, fishing out on a sandbar,
> hooks my joints
> and reels me back.

Now I'm at the phone trying to sound
composed; not like a person flailing.

The nurse consoles, a *hor*-rible drug,
letting the first syllable   balloon
like a bloated face; then, that maudlin caveat
meant to comfort: *Before steroids, half
the patients died.* For a moment, all I can think:

how odd
these phone chitchats
with strangers
about death.

There's no other drug?

> *Not for that.*

Other calls must be blinking on her phone
but she waits   waits

while I stall—treading water—until I can accept
until I can be grateful/be
eager for

that same drug/

higher dose.

Raynaud's Syndrome

A patriotic
salute to cold? My fingers
stiffen red white blue.

Medical Bills

White envelopes
pile up in drifts
upon the desk, unopened.

She knows what's required—
a pleasing manner and persistence—
to clear a path through their tangle
of errors, and settle on a sum
(or face a siege of dinnertime calls).

Each day, a relentless advance: more envelopes arrive.

Through their clear windows
her imprinted name
peeks out,

a reminder of—more than the money owed—
how vulnerable, how captive
she's become: waiting for results,
answers, a plan that will restore
her own self.

Full Lunar Eclipse, October

Out on the front porch to witness
Earth's sunset-red shadow
slide its slow caress
across a voluptuous moon,
the scent of late summer evening
not yet lost to frost,

outlooks realign.

Progress Notes

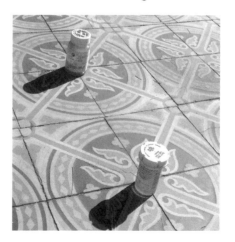

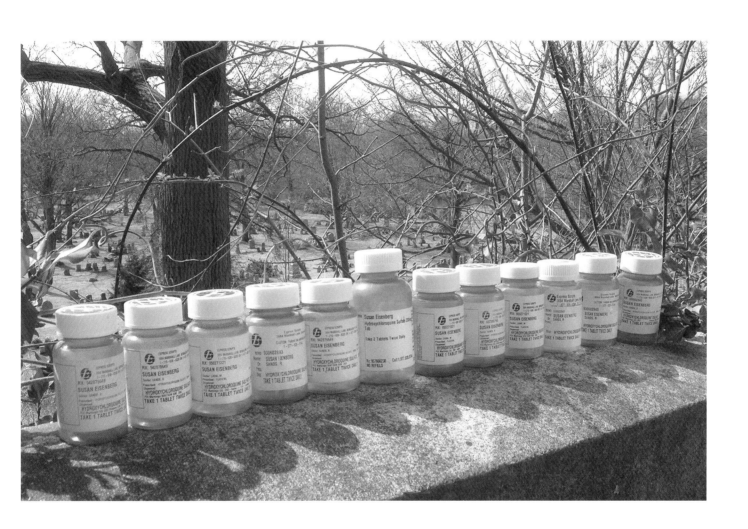

Would You Recommend Him?

He caught my body in freefall
and led me out from the cave
where I'd been cortisone's captive.

But I remember as keenly,
from our years of frequent appointments,
his exits:

how, framed in the exam room doorway,
he'd pause, turn back toward me
and—shoulders in a shrug—

deliver some news that electrified
the air
as I stumbled to dress.

Reading

I scan the new doc's face as she scans
my chart, waiting for—there!

that flash across her eyes—
what is it? sorrow?

For a moment, in this tiny way station,
dressed in the uniforms of our roles,

as she reads that one test result
written in neon

we're simply two humans
bobbing in fate's waters, hoping

no one drowns.
Her face turns toward mine:

professional,
composed.

Lab Test

I'll wait for *him,*
you almost say, as the skillful hands
you've had before guide someone else,
and a new tech pronounces your name.

Now you're sitting in *her* chair,
the arm rest flapped down locking you in,
sleeve up, soft inner elbow
exposed.

She asks your name and address. You
confirm name   and date of birth.
She nods, acknowledges the correction,
and counts out five vials.
Stiffen arm. A tap for the vein. Alcohol.
Tighten the fist

                    and turn away.

The needle enters smoothly. You breathe
and turn to watch the tube fill red.

That first vial's out. As she pops on the next,
you brace for the needle's whiplash.

Call Insurance Agent about
Your Balance: Lotsa $$$

All routine tests *are* fully covered, no cost to me,
she agrees. Then cheerily corrects
(I'm not the first) mistaken definitions.

> *routine* = preventative

> *preventative* = not due to any sign
> or symptom of illness or injury

While, true, I had no signs or symptoms,
and tests were meant to screen
for damage from a drug

and were (for me) routine,

that drug = evidence of illness.
I'll have to pay.

Dizzy

Like a helium balloon loosed
from a child's grasp

    my forehead
            floats up

my gaze follows

          and the ground
    starts to spin.

Explain *Lightheaded*, the Doc Asks

Instead of my head—
floating dots.

Her pen stays raised, I try again.

My head not solid. Only an outline.
Inside: a swarm of separate dots
drifting.

Her eyes tell me I am off-grid.

Now the doc gives a try,
pulls out her phrase book of standards
in her trained tongue,
her face hopeful I'll pick out a match.

     We press our palms
     against the same thick glass
     but can't make contact.

I shake my head. We move on.

My Daughter's First Year of Med School

As her syllabus probes the human body
system by system, I adjust to the rhythm.

Every three weeks: another organ
where dire lupus complications present.
Kidney. Heart. Lungs. Skin. Brain.
The phone rings.

Still alive, still mild. She knows.

But she needs to hear my voice,
press her stethoscope
against each syllable.

Appointment: MRI

I'm hardly eager to be locked in a box
with death's minions knocking about me
while the DJ in the sound booth intro's
avant-garde fusions
of truck horn, jack hammer, and timpani,
announcing playtime in minutes. But

I readied myself
(as best I knew how)
for Monday 7 PM.
Then gracefully adjusted
(even told a small joke)
to Wednesday 9 PM.

Then   Wednesday 8 PM.

Now once more they reschedule:
8 PM Thursday. A simple
                                twenty-
                                four-
                                hour
                                delay

lets loose a dambreak
of despair   foreboding.

The Technician Who Just Ran Your Tests
Pops Back in the Room / Asks a Tip-Off Question /
Disappears / Reappears Haiku

She'll sound nonchalant,
The doc wants to speak with you.
Steel yourself: bad news.

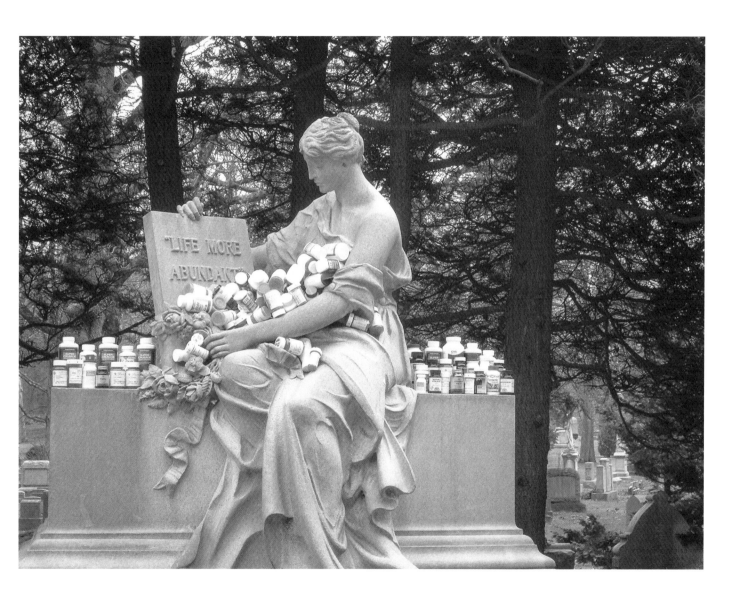

Emergency Triage

I smile at the mirror.   *All clear!*
Then check my eyes for droop—
Clear!—the sides of my face
as even as the nurse's voice
guiding my exam by phone,
propping me in a rescue hold
until we latch onto
                      a plan.

Emergency Appointment, Rheumatology

Face to face, we're upbeat,
calm, on task. Illness
only incidental to identity.

But glimpsed through glass, as she hurries back
to whatever caseload of heartbreaks
she interrupted
to examine me today,

the shoulders of her white coat sigh
with such sadness

I almost panic, follow after. I want
to reassure: tests just ordered
will show—not luck
losing ground—but nothing,
nothing at all. Her shoulders:

Not this one, too.

Scare

After years pecking each other,
my flock of illnesses and I set fencing
in place, become neighbors.

And then—4 AM!—with a shrieking screech,
a strange new one swoops in. Lightningstorms
ricochet
across the planes of my body. The breech
alarms the whole brood to squawking
and me to the floor, whining, *Isn't my glass full
to the brim? What about—*
(and here, I'm ashamed to say,
I shouted out names
and addresses. Yours. And, yours.)

The doc orders pricey tests and—
because she never mentions a name—
I suspect: That-One-I-Could-Not-Bear.

She mentions only its mark.
I surf the net, confirm the match. Fear swarms
from its hidden hive; the mind catapults
into preparations for what-
mightbemightbemightbeeeee.
My *end-this* options:
      A when money and pleasure run their course
      B when pain shouts, *Mercy!* or
      C upon results
just stop the pills. A final frieze.

A week passes. Haywire electrics taper.
Now the doc's on the phone with results.

Greetings exchanged calmly. And—

news is good! No explanation, but
symptoms have waned and Doom's ruled out
for now. Back to petty squabbles! Life.

Lupus Flare

I'm simply a serf.
Fatigue raises its scepter;
my eyes bow in sleep.

Bathing in Self-Pity

Those days when medical news plays the blues
I run a steamy tub, climb in, lean back and I'm
Nancy Kerrigan felled to the skating-rink floor:

clubbed knee hugged to my chest,
gold-medal face tear-streaked,
mouth open wide

wailing out to the deaf gods of fairness, *Why me?*
wailing out to the deaf gods of fairness, *Why me?*
wailing out, *Why me?*

until I can laugh
or the water's too cold.

Who Could Forget

such a simple thing
as taking pills
set out weekly
so predictably?
So it would seem. Yet

sometimes on Friday
there sit Wednesday and Thursday

quietly waiting,
like kids on porch steps
with their overnight bags long past
pick-up time,
while I've wished myself back
to a timebefore

until the body reminds.

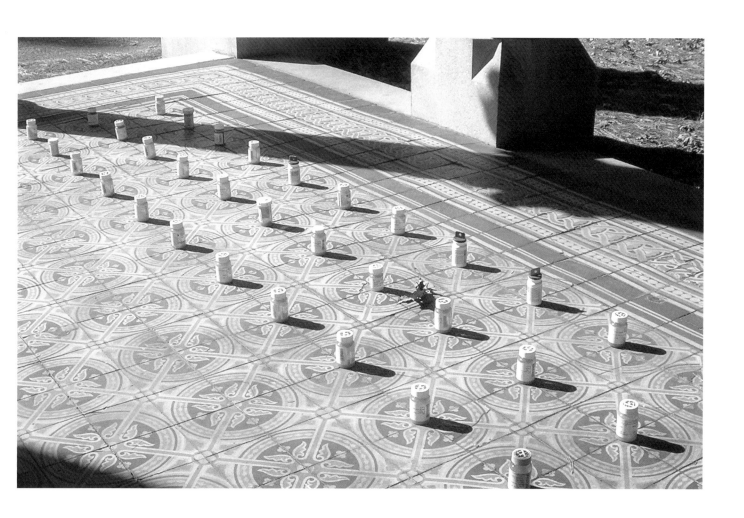

Friends and Enemies

Roast beets, 400 degrees.
A little oil, a little sea salt. About an hour.
Loosen from their skins. Good for the liver.

> Avoid dairy and red meat.
> Place protein at the periphery of your plate.

Carmelize brussel sprouts to unwrap
their savor. Cozy up to quinoa and tango
with turmeric: curry lentils, cauliflower, squash . . . .

> Avoid the sun. Shun alcohol. Serve
> divorce papers to sugar.

Marry wild mushrooms—all of them!—enokis
and shiitakes
and those meaty trumpets.

> Avoid the nightshades, provocateurs
> of the joints: eggplants, potatoes,
> and the tomatoes you planted in May,
> weeded and tended—now, ripe red
> in the garden, so round, so sweet . . . .

Family History

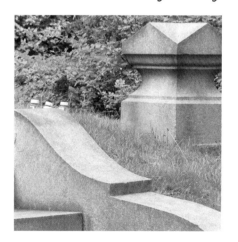

Early Lesson about Sick People

About the aunt for whom I was named
I was told just two facts.

    She died of diabetes.

    She was so fat,
    her hugs
    squeezed out your breath.

I never use that bad luck name.

Umbilical

1) Early Asthma Episode

A smiling med student with a clipboard
kneels beside our chairs at Urgent Care.
Calm as anyday, she asks me to rate
the health of my son—a wild stallion colt
of a boy—her earnest pen poised
to circle: excellent   good   fair   poor.

She's been assigned to fill in blanks
while we sit captive
in this narrow room waiting
for a rescue ladder to lift us
back to the known world.
My son is seven, but today—
his oxygen not sufficient
to buoy his body upright—
he let me carry him from the car
like a snowsuited toddler.

I don't remember what I said, only
how my son's full moon face
hung on my response.

2) Ten Years Pass
My son sounds the first alarm:
You've lost your strength.

Only after months, and more insistent signs,
do his words
assemble in my brain.
He keeps watch, points out each turn,
reminds me of the normal that was
his mom, leads me by the hand
through these cliffwalks he's scouted,
Are you okay? Are you okay?

In the 1950s

kept secret
until that still summer afternoon windows open
pear tree in full leaf: a cousin
kept almost in plain sight

that year that day asked
hours before dinner to sit at the table
for puzzles unpuzzled: why
at our aunt's home always
Play downstairs Stay downstairs
upstairs   where once I followed a ball—
Come back downstairs!—a folding screen
blocks a doorway   why

we learn: propped on pillows   a cousin our age
only grown-ups could see   a cousin with a name
our first hearing of her name

born perfectly gorgeous but
(solemnly explained) her head grew
grewgrewgrew   in the shape of a pear

my sister and I   10 and 7   imagine
and gigglegiggle—*Wicked!* my mother shouts
only wicked children would laugh shouts selfish brats
ashamed do not deserve should never have told

Oh dear Cousin PearHead Cousin NeverSeen
in dreams I swordfought like Zorro up that staircase
carried you to our pear tree
we brought you bracelets and ribbons

only children could see you

My Parents' Health Declines

One afternoon, when she ordered her husband of almost six decades to stand up straight, he stayed in a slouch. They immediately put on coats and drove to his doctor, who diagnosed a stroke and foretold imminent death.

Since her husband was the type to notice each morning whether he was alive or dead, and plan his day accordingly, the couple took their already-paid-for trip to Turkey (dismissing concerns of family who, as tactfully as they could, pointed out that, when it comes to dying, the familiar surroundings of home are preferable to somewhere so exotic). After Turkey, the couple traveled to Quebec, and then, London. Before each departure, doctors pointed to statistical charts and, after each return, shrugged. By now he was almost blind.

They continued their subscription to the theater, and monthly book discussion group. And he continued to drive, with her beside him shouting, *Stop sign! Red light! Car!!!* until the out-of-town daughter insisted that only the mother could drive—although the mother's eyesight also was failing. Luckily, the father was still a good navigator—he knew the streets that well—so he could, at the right moments, call out, *Turn left at the third traffic light,* and, *Not this street, at the next, take a right.*

But for spotting other cars, the blindness handicapped him. One day on the highway: CRASH! car totaled. An ambulance rushed them to the nearest emergency room. By good fortune, other than a few bumps and cuts, they were fine. But now without wheels. A friend in their apartment building, who understood from personal experience such imprisonment, wrote down the phone number of a very nice man who sold cars to seniors and repaired them after accidents. From him, they bought their first used car, and more than once required his repair services.

Only after the wife appeared in court for hitting a fire truck did she stop driving—against her husband's protests. *She just nudged it,* he insisted. And,

– 49 –

The fire truck was only a small one! Now, to get around, they were dependent on the kindness of their in-town daughter and those friends who still drove; and on the whims of the town's senior van whose schedule required a degree of patience for which the wife had never been known.

To the consternation of family and friends, the husband elected to have eye surgery that required a year for recovery. And then, expressed his determination to once again drive. Fortunately, the car had been sold back to the very nice man following the fire truck incident, saving the out-of-town daughter from having to say, *Absolutely not.*

They continued to do their own shopping. He held onto the cart for stability and slowly circumnavigated the store while she darted down each aisle they passed, grabbing groceries from the shelves and hurrying back to the cart before he reached the next aisle. They continued to go out to dinner at least once a week, though no longer to the fancier restaurants they once frequented. The wife, who had always glared at any less-than-fastidious behavior, acted as though she didn't notice her husband's public hiccups and burps, or the food he spilled on his shirt and pants. Rather than interrupting him as she always had, she seemed to have discovered his good company, and asked frequently for his opinion or requested he tell a joke, listening attentively as he grasped for words. They paid for everything by credit card; she had him sign the bill.

Meanwhile, doctors argued over which of his many ailments was most likely to win the line on his death certificate. Dismissing such nonsense, the wife told her husband that, at a year short of ninety, he was far too young to die. So he waited.

Past February, when the question of which sandwich he'd like for lunch could make him hang his head like a shamed puppy.

Past March, when the boundary between sleepandnap disappeared.

Past April, when an ambulance stole him from his wife's bed.

Past when he could dress himself, past when he could toilet himself, past when his swollen feet could steady his legs.

Into June, when he smiled only for ice cream and his wife.

Until July, when even she acknowledged it would be alright for him to leave her.

Meanwhile . . .

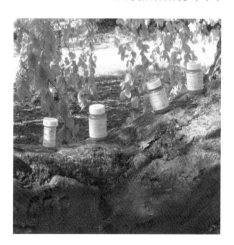

Malignant

Sly one, sixteen years you nested
in my bowtie gland—intimate
to each breath, swallow,
murmured sound—

outwitting countless pictures
and punctures until
you grew careless, or too big
to hide. Betrayed yourself:

not the well-mannered child,
but the playground tyrant.
Tell me, what seeds did you scatter
before you were cut out?

Cancer Survivor

What a weighty tag
to hang from one's neck
to be stamped
like a passport at border crossings:
1 year   5 years   10 years   20

as though the conjoined twins—
Lucky and Unlucky—could be cut apart;

as though the living
should separate

from those failures   the dead.

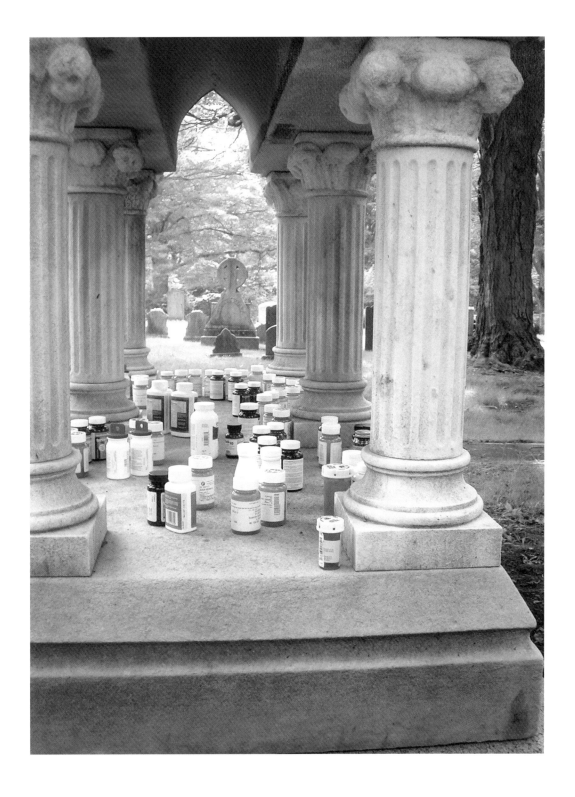

Waiting Room Etiquette

Check in. Take a seat & magazine.
I'm chill. Calm. Cocooned into
"Studies Explore Strategies for Staying Sharp."
Flip the page. Catch
in my sideview: a patient rise from her chair
and cross toward me. I burrow into the blur
of words, black on white. She crowds too close,
her weight shifting foot to foot, worry beads
tumbling from her mouth. Asks
about my tests: their danger.

She eavesdropped.
Stepped through my shield.
I will her
to return to her chair. I will her
to back herself across the room. I glare—
then see how fresh the scar across her neck

(a year behind my own):
I'm her placeholder.
She's looking for a postcard from the future.

From my purse I pick out two—
Centenarian Hoeing Her Garden,
and Boisterous Friends Bountiful Table—
and in my best script, across the back,
wish us both good luck.

A Puff of Dandelion Seeds Rides the Wind:
First CAT-Scan

Good luck,
says the doc
over the phoneline
and then
I'm propelled
into a cavernous
almost-empty room
and instructed
to remain motionless
while a moving conveyer
slides me
through the machine's spinning eye
to scan my insides for trouble.

Beneath the kind wish
danger hovers. Fists tense,
relax. In this sanctuary: only

myself   and this machine
transporting me into awareness
of luck   already pollinated.

The Doc Crunches Numbers

Multiplying the tumor's size
times my age, minus x, factoring in for y,
he spins a proof. Then calculates
in his head: 98th percentile! (my chance
at twenty more years)—*Death's
a drop-out.*

I'm tempted to argue,
remind him of the long odds
that landed me here: 20 to 1!
and I'm that one. Why trust
statistics now?

But the doc seems relieved,
so pleased to have good news,
I smile, too. Why not?

Tense

Had.
I had cancer.
I had surgery.
I had radiation treatment.
The cancer seems to be gone.
The cancer may be gone, but might return;
or, I may still have cancer, lurking unnoticed.
To announce myself *cured!* would court bad luck.
I may still have cancer lurking unnoticed.
Or, the cancer may be gone and return.
The cancer seems to be gone.
I had radiation treatment.
I had surgery.
I had cancer.
Had.

Raising Research Funds

Every disease needs its own colored ribbon
with matching handbag and walking shoes
to stand out in the crowd of hardships
and unluckies;

its own prancing show horse
to compete on the cocktail circuit.
An airbrushed celeb is always best. But even
an unknown—cheerful, photogenic, poised—
can open checkbooks
with the right family portrait
and beaten-so-many-odds tale
that highlights, in strong visual, triumph
over disease: an asthmatic track star,
an ice skating champ
with lupus, a prize-winning author with RA
who writes with her teeth.

History is full of such show-offs—
blind painters, deaf musicians—
rubbing their thumb in our one good eye.

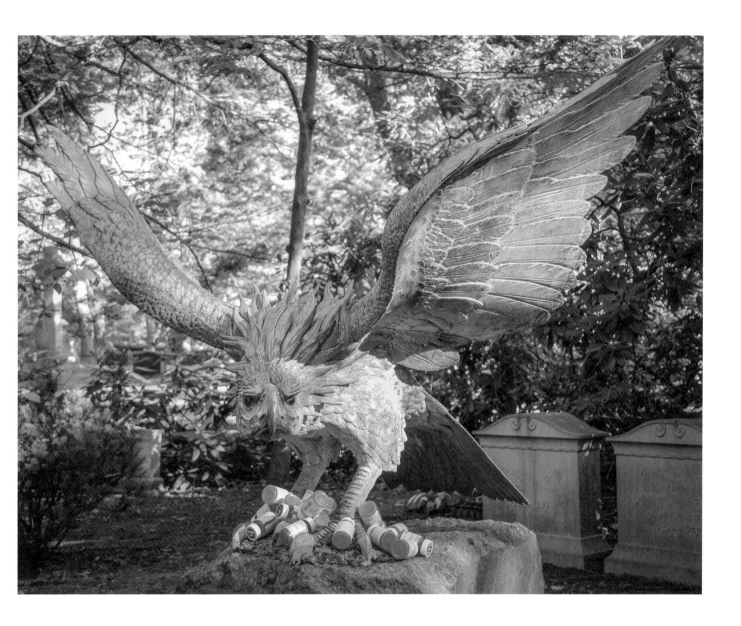

Patient Gallery Closed: Social Worker Explains

Gone. Had to. The whole program. *Hhwht!*
Too chaotic for a business like this. But I do
miss those artists,
their fervor swept us up.
Like a tsunami!—might have carried us out to sea
if not for Admin. Patients jumped aboard
but, let's say, the ship encountered turbulence.

I'm not defending Before: "each one huddled /
in the solitude / of his own fear. / No one speaks"
(one of their poems). But, honey, we had staff afraid
to call out a patient's name—such a howl
from the waiting room. One lady broadcasts:
    I'm about to find out if my eye damage
    from medication is permanent. Yes!
You should have heard the bloody fuss:
Sue them! Good luck, Sister! And crying!—
one for the other! as though each one
hadn't enough to cry for.

They'd get in with the doctors—and tick off
questions questions questions and go on and on—
like it's still the seventies! and no one's clocking time.

I hope you've seen the photo show up now: penguins,
ice formations. They had—imagine!
a patient comes in—frightened—and sees, *Headache*
(a carved head with pounded-in nails). Or,
a string of tiny paper pill cups called, *Daisy Chain:*
I'll Make It / I Won't. All that's down. Rules
are in place, guidelines. A great experiment,
but we can't risk complaints. We're a hospital,
a cheerful place.

Cancer Survivor Dies of Cancer

People, the patient we chose
for TV ads—whose story brings mega-hits
to our website and catapults profits—
died last night. We could

pull Paula's story from the web—
in the past, that's how we've handled
this kind of thing—but we can't
pull TV
without absorbing a huge loss, and can't
run the ads without Paula's videocam
on the web. It gets worse.

Her son's been calling, the family's quite upset.
I've had Jean take the calls: cool
things down, offer condolences, let them know
how much we all loved Paula. But
we'll need a decision today. The family
wants her story to stay up
with a new ending that they
write. And a photo
that's recent.

Our I'm-a-Survivor campaign
represents a major capital investment.
I've asked Marketing
to join us, give their angle.
And Legal.

Pancreatic

He'd never been shy to wish
extravagantly, or to kick
a deaf universe hard in the shins
for injustices large and small
documented in footnoted detail.

That was Before. And might be again

but Monday he wishes
simply
for results to be negative.

And, Tuesday, that the tumor
be operable.

Wednesday, that the tumor not be some reckless
adventurer, relentless explorer,
but a homebody
satisfied to sit quietly still.

Thursday, that the chemo be worth
its caravan of misery.
That he see another graduation. Or two.
And Rome with his wife. Not

grandchildren. Not golden
chosen retirement. Not a cure.
Modest wishes,
like the final matryoshka
that nests inside the larger dolls
and fits inside the palm.

Then Friday. *Oh!* Friday.

Terms

Doc-tor (from Latin: *to teach*). Beneath
this verbnoun's signature white coat
action rises in two snappy syllables led
by consonants of authority. One ends—
all business—with hard *c*; the other softens
into *r* before moving along on its rounds.

We want a mast that won't break in rogue waves,
experienced hands. It's the paired word
that's misnamed: *pa-tient*. Adjective cloaked
as noun, the word explodes, then retreats
into muffled sounds of the *acted upon*.
Defined by deference and willingness

to wait. Why? when I know investigators,
inventors, instigators. Dragon riders.

Hope

I offer my friend the green cocktail napkin
kept for weeks in my purse. Across

one corner, the name of a doctor, at work—
three thousand miles away—on a cure

for her brain cancer, jotted with borrowed pen
by someone met at a party. She accepts

the folded square, but bluntly discourages
more such notes: *There isn't anything.*

I'm chastened back to another friend's words,
in her thirtieth year of metastasis, midair

once again—between one chemo failing
and the next concoction—no trapeze bar

to grab: *We're always looking for hope
hope   that's not stupid.*

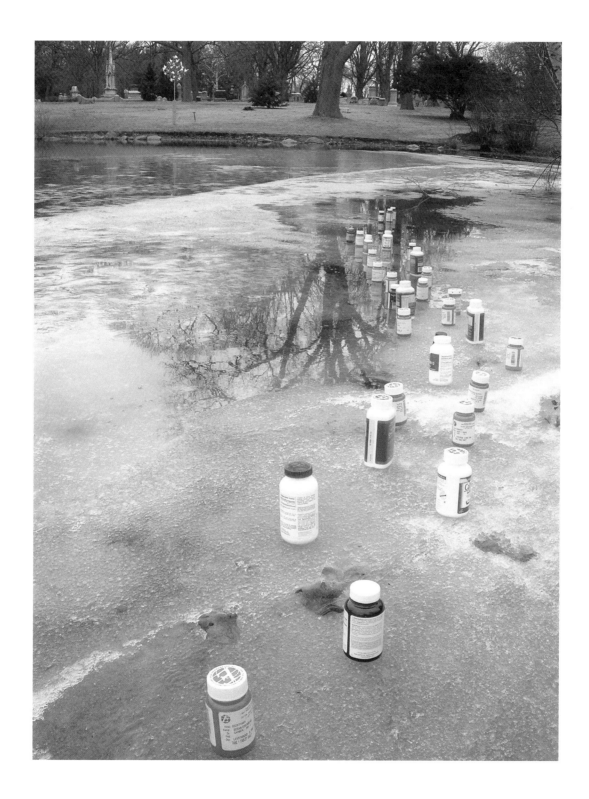

Notes

When diagnosed with lupus—and two years later, thyroid cancer—I was lucky to have Rita Arditti, a scientist and longtime activist in the breast cancer movement, as a close friend. Many of these poems grew or shifted from our wide-ranging conversations. The companionship and information-sharing of the lupus community have been invaluable, but I found a different freedom in talking across the balkanization of our illnesses, where the other person's difficulties or setbacks don't resonate so personally.

As someone who'd always relied on a healthy body, who'd performed physical theater and worked fifteen years as an electrician on union construction sites, the shift from *Health: Excellent* to *What's-going-on!?!* was a hard adjustment. I understood physical injury and brief illness, but auto-immune disease was new terrain.

"You'll be on this medication for the rest of your life," was the response when I asked how long I'd be on plaquenil. Empty prescription bottles began to accumulate, and multiply. I didn't know why I couldn't discard them, or what to do with them. I wanted to write—poems, or nonfiction—but couldn't find language, until I began to slowly find my voice and sense of humor in a cemetery.

I am fortunate to live near one of the country's earliest and finest Victorian cemeteries, evocatively landscaped for contemplative strolling. Walking in Forest Hills Cemetery one day, I imagined my empty medication bottles traipsing down the center of a carriage road. I asked Cecily Miller, then Director of the Forest Hills Educational Trust that sponsored innovative arts programming, for permission to create and photograph installations. She thought the project fit well with the Victorians' concept of cemeteries as places of reflection, and she generously shepherded the process. One photograph created an urgency for the next, until visual brought me to verbal.

The installation photos, for me, are visual poems. I've included poems alongside them at exhibitions, so it seemed natural to include some of the photographs alongside the poems.

Acknowledgments

Grateful thanks to the following publications in which poems first appeared: *Caduceus*: "Waiting Room Etiquette"; *The Examined Life*: "Lupus Outwits Me, Declares Martial Law"; *The Healing Muse*: "Explain *Lightheaded*, the Doc Asks"; *Hospital Drive*: "In the Beginning"; *Nimrod*: "My Parents' Health Declines"; *Off the Coast*: "Escape from Prednisone, Second Attempt," "Raising Research Funds," and "The Doc Crunches Numbers"; *Paterson Literary Review*: "Post-Diagnosis," "Disclosure," "Lupus Conference, Morningstar Baptist Church," "Scare," and "Umbilical"; *Salamander*: "Friends and Enemies"; and *Voices from the Porch* (Main Street Rag): "Full Lunar Eclipse."

Thanks to the New England Poetry Club for the Firman Houghton Award to "Medical Bills" and "Pancreatic."

Heartfelt gratitude to Forest Hills Cemetery and the Forest Hills Educational Trust, especially Cecily Miller, for their early support of this project; and to a project grant from the Puffin Foundation. For exhibition of photographs, thanks to Visual Aid, San Francisco; Kniznick Gallery, Brandeis University; Marran Gallery, Lesley University; Forsyth Chapel, Boston; and the Massachusetts Department of Public Health.

Deep thanks to the Lupus Foundation of New England and Women's Community Cancer Project communities, especially Denice Garrett, for their courage, research, wisdom and warmth; and to the support and encouragement of the Brandeis Women's Studies Research Center, and residencies at Hedgebrook.

Thanks to my very wonderful doctors for sharing their humanity and seeing mine; and for their patience for a poet's curiosity. Thanks to the Boston Medical Center Residency Program for their doctors' perspective on the poems and photographs.

For design and production of this book, and their caring midwifery, thanks to Estelle Disch, Denise Bergman, and especially Ilene Horowitz, Director of Font & Center Press.

And, most special thanks to my son and daughter, Simon and Zoe, who have been my teachers and healers.

About the Author

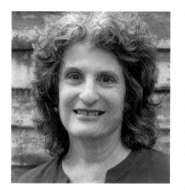

Susan Eisenberg, born and raised in Cleveland, Ohio, is a poet, visual artist, and oral historian, who works within and across genres. First introduced to the craft of poetry by Denise Levertov, she is a graduate of the MFA Program for Writers at Warren Wilson College, and taught for a decade at the University of Massachusetts Boston. She is author of three previous poetry collections—*Blind Spot*, *Pioneering*, and *It's a Good Thing I'm Not Macho*—as well as the nonfiction *New York Times* Notable Book, *We'll Call You If We Need You: Experiences of Women Working Construction*, optioned by MGM. Awards include a Mass Humanities "Freedom and Justice for All" grant and three residencies at Hedgebrook. A 35-year member of the International Brotherhood of Electrical Workers (IBEW), she was among the first women in the country to become a licensed union electrician. *On Equal Terms*, her 900-square-foot installation combining poetry with 3-D mixed media, audio, photography, found objects, and artifacts, has been exhibited in galleries in Massachusetts, Michigan, and New York. A longtime resident of the Jamaica Plain neighborhood of Boston, she is a Resident Artist/Scholar at the Brandeis Women's Studies Research Center where her projects focus on medical humanities and employment equity; and the 2016–2017 Twink Frey Visiting Social Activist at the University of Michigan.

CPSIA information can be obtained at www.ICGtesting.com
Printed in the USA
BVIW12n0000240516
449272BV00001B/1